Anti-Histamine Diet

Lower Histamine, Increase DAO, and Reverse Histamine Intolerance in Six Weeks

By

Anna Keating

D0391285

Anti-Histamine Diet: Lower Histamine, Increase DAO, and Reverse Histamine Intolerance in Six Weeks

ISBN-10: 1549737716

ISBN-13: 978-1549737718

Warning and Disclaimer

Every effort has been made to make this book as accurate as possible. However, no warranty or fitness is implied. The information provided is on an "as-is" basis. The author and the publisher shall have no liability or responsibility to any person or entity with respect to any loss or damages that arise from the information in this book.

Publisher contact

books@skinnybottle.com

A Thin Line

If you have been living inside your irritating, itchy little bubble, not knowing what causes your symptoms, except that it isn't an allergy that shattered your comfort, then chances are, you have been dealing with histamine intolerance.

The line between allergies and histamine intolerance is a thin one. If you have found yourself confused by the conflicting theories online, then worry no more, because this book is the only thing you need to put a stop to the uncomfortable symptoms you have been dealing with. Learn how histamine has been causing you all this trouble, as well as how to pull it by the root.

Let's deep dive into the essence of the amino acid called 'histamine', why we need it, how to know if we have too much of it, and what to do if your body can no longer degrade it. This book will provide you with the best histamine elimination diet, a 6-week meal plan, and in-depth insights that every histamine intolerant individual should read.

Still not sure if you are histamine intolerant? Why not join me on this irritation-free ride and find out?

ANNA KEATING

What is Histamine?

Just because people usually hear about this compound the unpleasant way, when doctors announce that they cannot quite tolerate it, that doesn't mean that histamine is not important to our overall health.

Histamine is a chemical, an active biological substance that can be found in almost every living organism. It is produced by the mast cells, and plays a very important part in the body's immune response.

Histamine is chemically classified as an amine formed as a result of the decarboxylation of the amino acid histidine. This extremely important compound was first discovered in 1910 in the plant fungus ergot. A year later, scientists also found that histamine was present in animal tissues as well. Think of histamine as the 'irritating' chemical. It is found in stinging nettles, and also found in the venom of many insects, such as bees and wasps.

Thanks to histamine, you itch and swell when you make contact with nettle's leaves. In the human body, histamine is found in almost every tissue, and most of it is stored as granules in the mast cells, as well as in the basophils and eosinophils, or otherwise known as the white blood cells. Once the histamine gets released from these granules, it immediately starts producing different effects (such as muscle contraction, blood vessel dilatation, gastric acid stimulation, etc.) within the body. But that's not the only reason why histamine is super significant for our overall health. It acts as a neurotransmitter, and is in charge of transferring chemical messages to the nerve cells.

If you still aren't impressed with what histamine means to our bodies, wait until you hear about its defending properties.

It helps the body to defend itself from invaders such as viruses, bacteria, or other harmful foreign bodies, hence why it is highly essential.

Additionally, in defending the body from harmful pathogens and being a huge part in any vital process, histamine also serves as the most important mediator in allergy symptoms, which means that in order to protect the body from this inflammatory reaction, the body must release histamine (as well as other anti-inflammatory mediators) to respond to the allergens.

To better understand the importance of histamine during an allergic reaction, let's look at this example. Imagine yourself having a picnic during allergy season in spring. You are sitting on fresh grass, surrounded with beautiful flowers. If you are prone to allergies, then you know what's about to happen. Not long after you start enjoying your time in nature you will start sneezing, your nose will start running, and you will suddenly become itchy. Have you ever wondered why this happens? And more importantly, what does histamine have to do with pollen allergy?

When something foreign like pollen enters your body, it triggers your immune system to respond to the foreign intruder. The pollen's microscopic grains, in this case, are treated as the enemy, and your body does its best to get rid of these attackers. In order to start the defending process, the body sends a signal to the mast cells and requests the release of its secret weapon – histamine.

The release of histamine to the site where the irritation has happened activates the proper response. This means that after, for example, your nose has been attacked by pollen, histamine stimulates the membranes to produce more mucus, and as a result, you will get a runny nose followed by a couple of sneezes. Chemically, histamine works only when bound to other receptors on the cells' surface. When histamine arrives at the irritation site, it does not cause one, but multiple important effects.

Probably the most important one is the effect of dilating the blood vessels, which is followed by swelling. This is the inflammatory response.   Have you ever been stung by a bee? The fact that the skin gets immediately puffy and round around the place where you got stung is thanks to the fact that histamine forces the blood vessels to dilate. And although we know how uncomfortable a bee sting can be, this inflammation response is how your body heals. Faster blood flow leads to the immediate delivery of white cells . The degree of inflammation in this case, or the allergic reaction that you will most likely experience in the pollen example, depends on how much histamine has been released, and this is something that varies from person to person.

Histamine works when it is bound to 4 receptors H1, H2, H3, and H4. In this, as well as in the majority of cases, histamine binds to H1, which is the most important of all receptors and is involved in allergic reactions.

Other Roles in the Body that Histamine Plays

Although we have already explained a few of the roles that histamine plays in the body, it would not do to shorten this section and rely on the few examples we have covered so far.

At first glance, histamine may seem like a not-so-important biological compound, given the fact that it's built with only seventeen atoms, but histamine is indeed essential for our body, and not only for the reasons we have talked about earlier in this chapter. The chemical properties that histamine has, allow it to be extremely versatile in binding, which is why it is involved in 23 physiological functions. It is super flexible and conformational, which allows it to easily interact.

Blood Pressure Decreases

Due to the fact that Histamine can force most blood vessels to dilate, it thus leads to a decrease in blood pressure. This is why people with high blood pressure often receive histamine intravenously.

Sleep – Wake Regulation

As was previously mentioned, histamine is a great neurotransmitter. Its cell bodies can be found in the hypothalamus (a portion of the brain in charge of many metabolic processes), from where the histamine neurons are projected throughout the brain in order to support wakefulness and lower symptoms of sleep. That is why the antihistamines are traditionally known to cause drowsiness (although the new ones are designed in a way that doesn't allow them to cross the brain and cause sedative effects).

Release of Gastric Acid

When bound to the H2 receptor, histamine can stimulate the parietal cells found near the stomach's gastric glands by supporting the acceptance of the water and carbon dioxide from the blood, and converting it to carbon acid. Inside the parietal cells, the carbon acid separates into bicarbonate and hydrogen ions, from where the hydrogen ions are pumped into the stomach's lumen, and bicarbonate ions once again diffuse into the bloodstream. When the stomach's pH levels start decreasing, the release of histamine is stopped.

Protection

When I say protection, I don't mean just defending the body from foreign invaders. Histamine is known to have some amazing effects that protect us from stress, drug sensitization, and convulsion. Histamine has also been discovered to have an effect on those mechanisms by which we tend to forget learned and memorized things.

Where Does it Come From?

I may have already said a word or two about where histamine is found in the body, but it is not the only place where it can be found. If you are wondering where histamine is found, here is a slightly more detailed explanation.

The Body Cells and Systems

Otherwise known as intrinsic histamine, histamine is present in all mammals – humans included – and serves the role of a biogenic amine. This type of histamine is produced when the enzyme histidine decarboxylase acts on the amino acid histidine (one of the twenty acids that make protein). Histidine decarboxylase can be found in cells that contain granules (such as mast cells and basophils). When the amino acid histidine comes in contact with the enzyme in these cells, it gets converted into histamine, and is stored in these cell structures waiting for a signal to be released. That is why histamine is present in the mast cells and basophils.

The Microorganisms in the Colon

Although the mast cells are where histamine is primarily stored, that is not the only place where it can be found. There are also a number of other microorganisms that can produce histamine. For example, there are a lot of bacteria in the human colon that are perfectly capable of producing histamine. How? The bacteria also produce histidine decarboxylase, and once protein with histidine content enters the large bowel and comes in contact with the enzyme histidine decarboxylase, it gets converted into histamine. Once there is histamine in the large bowel it can quickly and easily get transported through the bowel wall to many different parts of the body.

Natural Foods

Histamine is also present in a variety of natural foods, and this type of histamine which enters our body from an outside source is called extrinsic histamine. The microorganisms that convert histidine to histamine also exist in nature, and so, histamine can appear in our body from many outer sources. For instance, the fish gut is colonized by bacteria that produce histidine decarboxylase. Shortly after a fish dies, the bacteria in the gut begins to break down the tissue proteins while releasing histidine. This is the reaction that produces histamine. It is important to know that the longer the fish stays ungutted after it has been caught, the higher the level of histamine. In fact, the histamine levels can double every 20 minutes or so. Fish that are not gutted after being caught, such as shellfish, will continue producing histamine until the moment they become cooked.

There are also many foods that contain histamine or are known to have histamine-releasing properties.

Manufactured Foods

There are many food manufacturing processes that mostly rely on the production of all sorts of chemicals and amines for the sake of the flavor of the food. Many of these processes, especially fermentation, will produce a rather high amount of amines, and with them, histamine.

Histamine Intolerance

When people have an 'intolerance' it usually means that their bodies are sensitive to something. Take lactose intolerance for example. It simply means that the body cannot quite digest the natural sugar lactose, and therefore becomes extremely sensitive when milk or other dairy product is consumed. Histamine intolerance, on the other hand, means something different. Despite what the name suggests, when a person is histamine intolerant, it does not mean that they are sensitive and cannot tolerate histamine; it simply means that they have too much of it.

Like we said, histamine is an extremely important compound in our body that plays one of the key roles of keeping us healthy. However, when histamine levels pile up in the mast cells, histamine has a counter effect on our health. Excess histamine makes us feel sick.

In order for histamine to function effectively, and to fight foreign bacteria or viruses, it needs to be broken down. If our body fails to break down the histamine quickly or efficiently, it will begin to pile up in the mast cells. Think of it as a glass filled with water. Everything is fine until the water is below the top. You can lift your glass and drink it. But, if the water exceeds the top it is impossible not to spill it. The same goes for histamine. Everything is fine until your body has the ability to work with the histamine that has been stored inside your body. Once the histamine levels exceed your body's 'comfort zone', and your body can no longer use this compound efficiently, histamine intolerance occurs.

How Much is Too Much?

Now that we have mentioned that your body works fine until the histamine exceeds the levels which your body is comfortable functioning with, I am sure that you cannot help but wonder what the standard level is. How much histamine do you need to have piled up in your mast cells or basophils?

Generally, it is considered that levels of histamine between 0.3 and 1.0 ng/ml (nanograms per milliliter) in the plasma are normal. However, not everybody is built the same way and just because you, for example, have a histamine level that is higher than 1 ng/ml that doesn't mean that you will necessarily start experiencing symptoms. Some people are better at tolerating excessive histamine levels than others. However, that doesn't mean that having over 1 ng/ml of histamine in your body is healthy. Try to keep the levels within the normal range.

The Causes

There are quite a few physiological conditions that may lead to the occurrence of histamine intolerance:

Diamine Oxidase (DAO)Blocking

As previously discussed, the body first needs to break down the histamine in order for it to be able to travel to the irritation site and do its job. Under normal conditions, the histamine is broken down by two enzymes:

1.   N-Methyltransferase (HMT) which is in charge of breaking down the histamine inside the central nervous system.

2.   Diamine Oxidase (DAO) which is in charge of breaking down the histamine in the small intestine.

The latter is what has definitely received the most attention, since a deficiency of the DAO enzyme in the body can lead to histamine intolerance. If a person is DAO deficient, there will not be enough of this enzyme to break down the excess histamine levels that are either ingested through food or have been stored in the body. Unfortunately, DAO deficiency is the leading cause of histamine intolerance. And if you are wondering what may cause you to be DAO deficient, or to have something that blocks the DAO enzymes from doing their job, here is your answer:

-       The enzymes can be reduced as a result of an underlying gastrointestinal disease

-       There are certain types of medications that can cause the production and blockage of the DAO enzymes

-       People who regularly consume food high in histamine are prone to being victims of DAO dysfunction

-       There are also certain foods that block DAO

-       The consumption of certain foods that have the ability to trigger the histamine release, even if the food itself doesn't contain histamine. When the DAO enzymes are blocked and the histamine production is supported, dysfunction may occur.

Gastrointestinal Disorders

If you suffer from a certain gastrointestinal disorder, then chances are it is to blame for your histamine intolerance. Most people who deal with the following disorders become intolerant to histamine over time:

- Gluten Sensitivity

- Crohn's Disease

- Leaky Gut Syndrome

- SIBO (Small Intestine Bacterial Overgrowth)

- IBS (Inflammatory Bowel Disease)

- Ulcerative Colitis

Bacterial Overgrowth

Another thing that can cause histamine intolerance is the building up of the bacteria that is consumed through those foods that cannot be easily digested. The bacteria are known to produce histamine, and since it is in overgrowth, you can easily do the math and see that overgrowth bacteria = excess histamine. If your body produces way more histamine that the enzymes can degrade, you are not only a candidate for histamine intolerance but also many different allergies, as well as gastrointestinal disorders.

Allergic Reactions

When you have an allergic reaction, your body produces more histamine. This means that when you are experiencing an overreaction of your immune system to a particular substance, your body, in order to defend itself, will be forced to frequently request the release of histamine, which will result in a massive production of this compound.

Histamine, as we said, is beneficial during allergy season as it helps the body defend itself, but when you are allergic to something and you expose yourself frequently to that substance (without knowing that you are allergic) you can also cause a disbalance in your histamine levels, and eventually become intolerant to it. The best treatment, in this case, is to avoid the allergy, which triggers the stop of excessive histamine production.

There are also some rare cases, usually when there is a drug, venom, or food allergy, where the entire body is forced to produce a massive amount of histamine which leads to anaphylactic shock, which is mostly life-threatening. This is followed by difficulties in breathing, wheezing, nasal congestion, abdominal pain, coughing, anxiety, and a faint pulse.

UV Light

Believe it or not, many studies indicate that UV light is also among the common causes of histamine intolerance. UV light triggers the release of histamine, and if exposed to it frequently, you have a high chance of becoming histamine intolerant over time.

Certain Medications

Studies have also shown that histamine intolerance may also be caused by phenothiazine compounds that are usually found in medications prescribed for treating psychiatric conditions from anxiety to schizophrenia. However, many over-the-counter drugs can also cause disruption in histamine balance and block the DAO enzymes. Anyone who is on the medications below and experiencing some 'allergies' should check for histamine intolerance:

-       Immune Modulators (Enbrel, Humira, Plaquenil)

-       Non-Steroidal Anti-Inflammatory Drugs (Aspirin and Ibuprofen)

- Antidepressants and Antipsychotics (Zoloft, Prozac, Cymbalta, Effexor)

- Antiarrhythmics (Norvasc, Cardizem, Metoprolol, Propranolol)

Other not so common causes

- High-intensity exercises in a warm environment

- People with periods of high estrogen levels

- High levels of stress can also decrease the ability of the enzymes to degrade the histamine in the body

The Symptoms

When there is an excessive amount of histamine built up in the mast cells, the body is unable to break it down efficiently, and so, a range of symptoms may appear. Know that most of the symptoms on the list below are also symptoms of allergic reactions. Make sure to check if you are perhaps histamine intolerant if you experience these symptoms:

- Anxiety

- Abdominal Cramps

- Sinus Problems

- Tissue Swelling and Inflammation

- Dizziness

- Vertigo

- Acid Reflux

- Digestive Disturbances

- Hypertension or Hypotension

- Sneezing

- Itching

- Temperature Dysregulation

- Breathing Problems

- Abnormal Menstrual Cycle

- Conjunctivitis

- Headaches or Migraines

- Trouble to Fall Asleep

- Vomiting

- Hives

- Tachycardia

- Fatigue

- Flushing

The Complications

Histamine travels throughout the bloodstream and gets transferred to every part of the body. This is extremely useful when we need an immediate immune response to defend us from foreign bodies, but not so much when you have piled up histamine. Because of the fact that it travels throughout the body, histamine can easily affect our brain, skin, gut, lungs, as well as our entire cardiovascular system. When we have piled up histamine in our body, this can contribute to the occurrence of some hazardous conditions.

If left untreated, histamine intolerance can cause a broad range of complications:

Osteoporosis

Most of the cells that are in charge of releasing histamine are extremely important to our bone health. When we have excess histamine levels these cells become unable to function properly and this can further lead to osteoporosis. In fact, experts suggest that inhibiting the mast cells may actually treat osteoporosis.

Brain Degeneration

When histamine is piled up in the brain, it can easily damage the neurons through inflammation. This can lead to brain degeneration and even Parkinson's disease. A study performed on patients with Parkinson's disease showed that the patients were unable to degrade histamine in the brain.

Cancer

Recent studies have found a strong link between excess histamine and cancer. Studies suggest that histamine and mast cells promote and inhibit cancer. Probably the greatest discovery regarding the histamine and cancer link is the fact that melanoma skin cancer is actually stimulated by histamine, based on lab tests.

Multiple Sclerosis

It has been scientifically proven that histamine receptors are indeed involved in the occurrence of multiple sclerosis; some of them promote the disease, while others inhibit it.

Meniere's Disease

Chronic dizziness, hearing loss, and tinnitus that appear as a result of this disease are symptoms that can be caused by an excessive amount of histamine in the body.

Disease Vulnerability

Histamine has the tendency to increase the penetrability of the barrier of the blood and brain. When you have high histamine levels, they significantly affect the barrier and can leave the door open for many bacterial infections and other diseases to swoop in. Note that the disruption of the blood-brain barrier contributes to the development of Alzheimer's disease, multiple sclerosis, epilepsy, and meningitis.

Histamine and Other Conditions

Besides the fact that high levels of histamine can cause certain illnesses to occur, it can also worsen many already existing conditions. If you are struggling with some of the conditions above, here is why it is of the utmost importance that you bring balance to your histamine levels as soon as possible:

Histamine and Hormones

Women already have a lot to deal with when those hormonal periods come knocking on their door, but being histamine intolerant and hormonal, now that is a combination you need to be aware of. Histamine levels tend to oscillate along with the hormones (mostly estrogen) at ovulation. If you are histamine intolerant, the symptoms of this condition may worsen during ovulation.

On the other hand, pregnant women experience relief in this symptom during pregnancy, since their placenta produces a great number of DAO enzymes. However, after giving birth, unfortunately, the symptoms of histamine intolerance return.

Histamine and Eczema

Eczema, medically known as atopic dermatitis, is an inflammatory condition of the skin that can be irritating. If you suffer from this condition and you have been experiencing worse symptoms and severity of your eczema, it may be as a result of being histamine intolerant, which worsens the condition.

Histamine and Anaphylaxis

Studies have shown that the majority of people who are vulnerable to severe allergic reactions, also known as recurrent anaphylactic reactions, are most likely victims of histamine intolerance, as well. This combination of severe allergies and histamine intolerance can be life-threatening.

Testing for Histamine Intolerance

Unfortunately, unlike most conditions, there aren't any proven tests that can successfully show whether a person is definitely histamine intolerant or not. The most common way of testing for histamine intolerance is by taking the DAO test, which shows whether the DAO levels are normal or not. However, this is definitely not a full proof method, since it isn't just the DAO enzymes that can degrade histamine. It is possible for levels of DAO not to be as disrupted, and still, the person can have a histamine intolerance.

The 23andme genetic test that looks at the production of DAO enzymes is another way of testing, however, also not very successful. Sure, when a person has a homozygous mutation, they will most likely be histamine intolerant, however, this usually does not happen until after the person's gut barrier gets broken down and the adrenal glands can no longer keep up with the demands. This usually happens after a very stressful period in that person's life has passed. So, most of you can cross this one off your list.

Another experimental method is the skin-prick test. It is promising since in a test study, 79% of those who were histamine intolerant reacted to the test. However, the test doesn't show either the enzymes, or the ingestion of high-histamine foods, and let's be honest, there is a 21% chance that the test will be incorrect, which is not a number that you should rely on when doing the test.

So, what can you do in order to be sure whether you are histamine intolerant or not? First of all, you need to evaluate related disorders and conditions such as allergies, gastrointestinal disorders, etc., but if you still have doubts even after evaluating the related symptoms, the best thing you can do is try the elimination diet, from this book. As proven by many experts, this diet is the best test plus treatment for histamine intolerance. You eliminate all of the histamine-rich foods from your diet, and keep track of your progress for some time. If the symptoms improve after some time, then you are probably histamine intolerant. If not, consult with your doctor to do some more tests in order to determine the real culprit.

Diagnosing Histamine Intolerance

According to recent research, histamine intolerance occurs in approximately 3 % of the population, and in 20 % of these cases occurs when histamine-rich foods are consumed in combination with some DAO inhibitors (like alcohol). 80 % of the histamine intolerant are women.

As I said in the previous section, unlike other conditions, histamine intolerance is pretty hard to diagnose. Not only the factors that have been considered, but also a reliable test to check for histamine intolerance, has not been invented because many doctors are unaware of histamine intolerance as a condition. This might be a result of a small number of people who suffer from it.

The point is, although we live in a world where there is advanced medicine, not every clinician will consider histamine intolerance as a contributing factor to the patient's health problems.

In addition, a healthy diet containing histamine-rich foods is recommended, which would be great for those who have normal values of histamine, but threatening for those who are histamine intolerant.

In short, histamine intolerance remains a condition that in many cases is left undiagnosed and therefore untreated. If you suspect that you are histamine intolerant and have the symptoms from before, please, contact your doctor as soon as possible and let him know that you believe you are histamine intolerant. If all tests suggest otherwise and you still remain struggling with the same symptoms, take the matter into your own hands and try the anti-histamine diet from this book.

Histamine Intolerance vs Food Allergies

Since the symptoms are very similar, histamine intolerance is, in most cases, mistaken for a food allergy. But the truth is, as similar as they appear, these two conditions are actually quite different.

A food allergy is a hypersensitive immune reaction when there are IgE (Immunoglobulin E) antibodies produced against a certain allergen (in this case a type of food protein). When the person who is sensitive to a certain type of food ingests it, the body immediately releases inflammatory mediators (histamine included). This usually happens a couple of minutes after the allergenic food has been consumed. The allergy symptoms appear immediately after consumption, regardless of how small the food quantity.

The symptoms of histamine intolerance, although they greatly resemble allergic symptoms, does not occur immediately after a histamine-rich food has been consumed. This is because the histamine in the body needs to first reach a certain, critical, level so that the tissues can start responding. Additionally, a small amount of histamine, unlike a small amount of allergen food, does not matter for the occurrence of the histamine-intolerance symptoms. It is the overall amount of histamines in the body that matters. Just like the example with the glass of water. It is okay until the glass becomes so full that the water ends up spilled all over the floor. It is the overall level of histamines that matter.

If you think you have an allergic reaction, test yourself. If skin and blood tests come back negative, you might want to consider the fact that it happened because you are histamine intolerant. Histamine intolerance is not mediated by the antibodies from the IgE type, so these types of tests are not accurate for this condition.

Is Histamine Intolerance Treatable?

Once you realize that you suffer from a certain condition, the first thing that, naturally, comes to mind is how to treat it. The good news about histamine intolerance is that you can definitely treat this hazardous condition and bring balance back to your gut and liver.

Unlike an allergy, that cannot be treated, only soothed, you can lower your histamine levels and go back to your old (okay, slightly healthy) menu.

But is it for good? Upon my research, I have realized that apart from wondering whether it is treatable, people also want to know if they can treat it for good. The answer is, of course, yes, but under what conditions?

I would want nothing more than to tell you that once you regulate your histamine levels you can dive straight back into a bowl of high-histamine food, but that would be a lie. You see, not everyone becomes histamine intolerant for the same reasons, and for some people, it is in their genes to not be able to successfully degrade histamine. These individuals should be careful about what they eat even after they heal their gut and lower the histamine levels. Of course, that doesn't mean that they will never be able to enjoy frozen yogurt again, but merely do it with great caution and strive not to experience the histamine intolerance symptoms again.

As to how you treat histamine intolerance, read on to find out.

Choosing the Right Anti-Histamine Approach

If you have been struggling with histamine intolerance as a result of, for example, some medication that you used to take, the solution here is actually quite simple, and in this case, the histamine intolerance can not only be easily diagnosed, but easily reversed, as well.

However, for some people, the treatment is not that simple. Most people mainly depend on their antihistamine diets in order to reverse the intolerance and lower their histamine levels.

You have a couple of options that you can use to try regulating histamine levels:

DAO Supplements

For some people, histamine intolerance happens purely as a result of the disrupted DAO enzymes, and most of them can easily regulate this by taking DAO supplements and not making any drastic changes to their diet, except trying not to ingest too much histamine that may interrupt the treatment. This is not by any means the healthiest nor the cheapest option, however, many people found this approach to be quite helpful. If the DAO enzymes are the only thing that has been causing you problems, consult with your doctor in order to start taking the supplements.

Low-Protein Diet

As previously discussed, histamine is mainly made from amino acids. And since these amino acids are derived from protein, it is logical that foods high in protein can affect the histamine levels. This is especially the case with food protein that cannot be easily digested in the gut, since the levels of histamine are known to increase as the food is digested. Because it is digested slowly and is left to age in the gut, this feeds bacteria, which only feeds the hazardous circle.

Elimination Diet

Elimination is, by far, the best treatment for histamine intolerance, and it is the type of diet that we will focus on in this book. So what exactly is the elimination diet? The elimination diet, as the name suggests, is eliminating all foods that are high in histamine, and relying only on safe, low-histamine food choices that will not worsen the symptoms.

How does it work? The elimination diet eliminates all histamine foods from the individual's diet for a certain period of time, usually between one and three months. So, for that period of time (in our case that would be 6 weeks) the person is not allowed to consume any histamine-rich foods. During this time he or she will track the progress and see if the symptoms indeed improve. If so, the person can then start slowly reintroducing these types of foods, one by one and in moderation, so that he or she can spot any changes and see what types of food their body can tolerate, and what not. After that, they can see what types of food they can and cannot enjoy in the long term.

Studies have found that this diet is the best choice for diagnosing, as well as for treating histamine intolerance.

Cutting Back on Histamine

Avoiding histamine completely is simply impossible since almost every type of food contains some amount of this compound. The important thing is to avoid foods that contain a higher amount of histamine. However, that is easier said than done.

The elimination diet is not like a low carb diet. You cannot simply read the food label and know how much histamine a certain food contains. Unless, you own a lab, it is pretty impossible to determine exactly how much histamine is in a food. And that isn't even the trickiest part. What's even more challenging is the fact that histamine levels in food are known to vary. For instance, a freshly-caught tuna fillet is very low in histamine and therefore safe to eat, but a small can of tuna can range from 0 to over 40 mg/kg.

But wait, before you announce a hunger strike. There are general guidelines that can help you select exactly which foods you should and shouldn't put on your dinner table.

Histamine-Rich Foods to Avoid

Here are some foods that contain a high amount of histamine, and therefore should be eliminated from your diet:

Milk

If you spend some time online, searching for what is safe to eat for a histamine intolerant person, you will come across many split theories about whether plain milk is safe to consume or not. Although there are people that suffer from histamine tolerance but still tolerate milk, I suggest you avoid complicating your condition with milk, when there are so many other yummy substitutes.

Fermented Products

Fermented products are probably at the top of every histamine-rich food list. Make sure to steer clear from:

-        Yogurt

-        Butter

-        Ripened and Aged Cheese (cheddar, goat cheese, feta, brie, blue cheese, Colby, etc.

-        Buttermilk

-        Kefir

-        Soy Sauce

-        Sauerkraut

-        Vinegar

-        Kombucha

Nuts

Nuts, especially walnuts, cashews, and peanuts, are known to spark controversy among nutritionists. Some will tell you that they are high in histamine, but that is actually not true. Nuts do not contain histamine, but *histadine*. Histadine is actually an amino acid that some gut bacteria uses to produce histamine. Now, this doesn't mean that you should avoid eating peanut butter altogether, however, keep in mind that nuts CAN raise the histamine levels for some people. If you are a fan of the "Better safe than sorry approach", keep nuts away from your anti-histamine diet.

Gluten

It is important to avoid gluten because of its ability to cause permeability in the intestines, which will result in a 'leaky gut'. And since keeping the gut healthy during histamine reversing is as important as avoiding high-histamine foods, gluten should, therefore, be crossed off your grocery list.

Yeast

Despite the fact that it does not actually contain histamine, yeast is, in fact, a catalyst for histamine generation in manufacturing. This may be tricky if you are a bread-lover, but there are tons of yummy gluten-free and yeast-free breads and baked goods that you can buy in the supermarket. If not, there is always the option of preparing them yourself.

Processed and Cured Meat

Salami, sausage, bacon, prosciutto, and jerky may be yummy, however, they are also packed with histamine. Make sure not to include any cured or processed type of meat on your anti-histamine menu.

Fish and Shellfish

Mahi-mahi, mackerel, sardines, tuna, anchovies, and herring should all be avoided. You should also make sure not to eat any canned, smoked, or pickled fish. When it comes to shellfish, that food group is absolutely off limits. Like we already said, they are not gutted, and therefore very high in histamine.

Vegetables

Although our mothers were right, forcing us to eat our veggies, when you are histamine intolerant, the veggies-are-healthy rule does not apply to all types of vegetables. You may be surprised with this list :

- Spinach

- Eggplant

- Olives

They are high in histamine and therefore should be eliminated from your diet.

Tomatoes may not be rich in histamine, but they are known to be histamine-releasing because they trigger the release of histamine after consumption. They should also be avoided. Needless to say, but that also goes for tomato paste, ketchup, pasta sauces, etc.

Pickled vegetables, well, anything that has been pickled in general, is also not allowed in the anti-histamine diet.

Mushrooms can be eaten from time to time, in moderation.

Fruits

Although some of these may contain some amazing properties, they are either high in histamine or they trigger the release of histamine and should be avoided:

- Avocados

- Strawberries

- Papaya

- Citrus Fruit

- Pineapple

- Banana

- Raspberries

- Guava

Dried foods (raisins, and dates included) are generally considered high in histamine and shouldn't be consumed.

Some people say that they are also intolerant of kiwis, pears, and grapes, however, I have found that most people tolerate them well, and they are not that high in histamine, so feel free to consume them in moderation.

Chocolate

I am sorry, but this guilty pleasure is known to trigger the release of histamine and should be crossed off your dessert section in your menu.

DAO Blocking Foods

There are some types of food that block the DAO enzymes. Make sure not to consume these ingredients:

- Alcohol

- Energy Drinks

- Green Tea

- Black Tea

- Mate Tea

Other things that you should absolutely avoid are:

- Sweets with preservatives

- Ready meals

- Artificial coloring

- Some spices like cinnamon, curry powder, chili powder, nutmeg, cloves, anise

Safe Food Choices

Now that you know what types of food should be avoided, it is time to learn what the safe choices to consume are. Below you will find foods that are generally considered to be low in histamine and can therefore be incorporated into your anti-histamine diet.

Meat

You can eat meat as long as it is fresh. Beef, poultry, pork, and lamb are all welcome, as long as it hasn't been refrigerated for a long time.

Gluten-Free Grains

Grains that do not contain gluten can be safely enjoyed during the elimination diet. That includes:

- Rice

- Quinoa

- Oats

- Millet

- Buckwheat

- Corn Grits or Polenta

Fish

When you are histamine intolerant, eating fish can be a true challenge. Is it safe enough? Is it fresh enough? The best answer is – eat fresh fish that you have caught yourself or you bought from a reliable fish market. I strongly recommend you find yourself a local fisherman that you will explain your condition to, and who will sell you only freshly caught and gutted fish. This is in case you cannot go fishing yourself, which is always a better option. Fish that have been gutted within half an hour after being caught, are considered to be low in histamine and safe to eat.

Eggs

When it comes to eggs and histamine, you will also come across many conflicting theories. If you have done some research, then you would have likely noticed that some people dump eggs in the safe-to-eat group, while others think they belong to the histamine-release category. The truth is, eggs are perfectly safe to eat as they are low in histamine. Then why all the confusion? It is true that egg whites tend to trigger the release of histamine, but only in their raw form. Cooked eggs are not only safe to eat, but also recommended by all experts. Make sure to eat them hard boiled and well cooked.

Dairy Substitutes

Coconut milk, hemp milk, almond milk, rice milk, and coconut oil are all recommended by specialists, as they contain a low amount of histamine.

Young Cheese

Cheeses that haven't matured and haven't been processed are low in histamine and safe to consume. They include:

- Cream Cheese

- Ricotta Cheese

- Cottage Cheese

- Mozzarella Cheese

- Mascarpone

-     Curd Cheese

Fruits and Vegetables

All fruits and veggies that haven't been mentioned in the forbidden group from before, are generally safe to consume.

Olive Oil

Olive oil is welcome to the elimination diet so feel free to use it not only for cooking but for drizzling over salads and food whenever you like.

Leafy Herbs

Try to flavor your meals with leafy herbs instead of adding spices. They are not only low in histamine but most of them actually have the ability to bring balance back to your mast cells.

Histamine-Lowering Foods

Yes, you read that right. There are actually certain types of fruit that are not only low in histamine and safe to consume, but they will also help you fight off inflammation faster, and stabilize your mast cells. Once the mast cells become balanced, the histamine lowering will occur naturally. And the best part is that there isn't a single ingredient from the list below that you will not find absolutely delicious.

Apples

Who doesn't like apples? And if apples are about to help you break down the histamine levels the natural way, then dig in. Eat them fresh, juice them, add them to your smoothies, salads, and even bake some gluten-free yummy pies with them. Just make sure not to peel them since the nutrients are mostly found in their skin. Many studies have recommended them as being capable of inhibiting the histamine release.

Black Rice Bran

If you thought that brown rice was the healthiest, then think again. Studies have shown that black bran rice not only has multiple benefits for your overall health, but it can also prevent the release of histamine from mast cells. Brown rice, on the other hand, is not that beneficial for you.

Ginger

This rhizome is known to be a great inhibitor of allergic reactions, and can also help you lower your histamine levels. Ginger has been traditionally used like an H2 inhibitor, however, a study from 2009 concludes that ginger is also an amazing mast cell stabilizer.

Nettle

A 2009 study suggests that nettle is also a great mast cell stabilizer, but that's not all. It also has the potential to lower histamine by working at the receptor H1. And although it is mostly consumed as a tea, nettle leaves can also be incorporated into your diet in many different ways. Soups and smoothies are some great suggestions.

Turmeric

Besides giving your meals amazing taste and color, turmeric is also packed with the most amazing properties. But besides its ability to relieve inflammation and enhance body cleansing, turmeric can also inhibit mast cell activation. A word of advice: freeze its rhizomes and grate them over your dishes. It will give them a great cheddar-like flavor.

Thyme

Thyme is more than just an amazing flavor for your dishes. Its powerful combination of high vitamin C content and flavonoids also contributes to histamine lowering and mast cell stabilizing. Plant some in your garden so you will never run out of fresh Thyme.

Onion

Onions are incredible prebiotics that can bring balance back to your gut in an instant. It has not only been concluded that onions can inhibit the release of histamine from the mast cells, but they also lower the levels in blood plasma.

Garlic

Famous for its antioxidant properties, garlic also serves as an amazing prebiotic. But besides regulating your gut, studies also show that garlic can contribute to the decrease of the histamine levels in the body.

Holy Basil

Minty, floral, and naturally sweet, holy basil is a very versatile herb that can be used in almost all dishes, mostly in pasta and salads. Holy basil is known to be a great adaptogen, but its histamine releasing properties are what interests us the most at the moment. Apart from using it fresh, you can also contribute to histamine lowering by drinking dried holy basil tea.

Peach

Peach cobbler anyone? This juicy summer fruit is not only sweet and one of the most delicious fruits, but it is also healthy. Studies show that peaches have the ability to inhibit the allergic inflammation derived from the mast cells.

Mung Bean Sprouts

A study from 2016 found that mung bean sprouts are not only healthy, but they also offer an amazing protection against the degranulation of the mast cells. Being high in flavonoids, they also support the process of breaking down the histamine.

Capers

Besides adding a peppery taste to your dinner, capers can also help you say goodbye to histamine intolerance. They are not only packed with anti-inflammatory, anti-oxidative, and antiviral properties, they also possess antihistamine properties. Please note that we are talking about fresh capers only. Preserved capers are neither anti-histaminic nor low in histamine.

Pomegranate

This jewel-like sweet and tart fruit contains polyphenols and is really high in antioxidants. But the best part of all is its ability to stabilize the mast cells and prevent histamine release.

Peppermint

Mostly used like an H2 antagonist, peppermint provides an amazing effect for allergic rhinitis. It is also packed with flavonoids, which greatly hinder the release of the histamine from the mast cells. Do not drink peppermint tea only. Use it fresh in salads, smoothies, pasta, etc.

Chamomile

It may help you fall asleep better at night, but that is not the only thing that chamomile tea can do for you. A study from 2011 has found a strong link between chamomile and obstructed histamine release. Try to use fresh flowers over dried ones whenever possible, as they are much healthier.

Watercress

Being part of the cruciferous vegetable family, watercress is the perfect addition to your salad which will add an amazing tangy and peppery taste. If you enjoy eating watercress, then you probably love the fact that watercress is actually able to inhibit an amazing 60 % of the histamine from the mast cells.

Tarragon

Being one of the most powerful antioxidants among herbs, there is no doubt about the benefits that tarragon can contribute to your overall health. Besides adding an anise flavor to your meals, this amazing herb is also a great stabilizer for mast cells.

Pea Sprouts

Pea sprouts contain a great amount of DAO enzymes that can help with the degradation of your extra-cellular histamine. And while almost every member of the Fabaceae family contains diamine oxidase, pea sprouts hold the crown with the highest concentration of DAO.

Galangal

Galangal, or otherwise known as Thai ginger, is amazing at preventing anaphylaxis, as well as for regulating the mast cells. Its delicate flavor can be easily added to your meals after a trip toAsian grocery stores.

Nigella Sativa

Also known as : black cumin, onion seeds, Roman coriander, and fennel flower, both the oil and seeds of nigella sativa will defend your gastric mucosal layer and offer some amazing antioxidant properties. Besides, it will give your dishes a great bitter, and oregano-like taste.

Supplements for Histamine Intolerance

If you or your doctor think that your balanced diet and regular consumption of histamine lowering foods are not enough for you to successfully reverse your histamine intolerance, or if you have food allergies and cannot eat any important food groups, then taking a supplement is perhaps the smartest choice.

There are a lot of supplements that can be taken with the purpose of preventing the release of histamine, however, please do not take them without consulting your physician. This is especially important if your doctor has prescribed you medications, as some supplements tend to interfere with certain drugs.

Copper

Copper deficiency has been associated with histamine intolerance, and since this micronutrient can also increase the levels of the DAO enzymes, taking copper as a supplement is definitely something that you should discuss with your doctor.

Probiotics

Now this is something that I highly suggest. Like I already said, a healthy gut is something that should be as important to you as focusing on breaking down your histamine levels, because if there are unhealthy bacteria in your gut you will never be able to regulate your histamine levels. And probiotics will provide you with just that.

When choosing probiotics to include in your diet, keep in mind that it isn't the genus that's important, but the strain. Speaking of beneficial probiotics, here are the probiotic strains that you absolutely need to incorporate into your balanced diet:

Bifidobacterium Longum – Keeping your gut balanced and preventing the growth of harmful bacteria, this probiotic strain is an absolute must.

Bifidobcterium Infanitis – As the name suggests, this strain is especially beneficial or babies. If you are pregnant, you might want to supplement your diet with this probiotic strain in order to pass some good bacteria to your little one.

Lactobacillus Rhamnosus GG – This is probably the safest and most-researched probiotic strain that you can include in your diet. It will stimulate your immune system and actually degrade the histamine.

Lactobacillus Salivarus - Another powerful histamine degrader that should be a part of your anti-histamine diet. This probiotic strain will definitely not trigger any unpleasant symptoms.

Lactobacillus Plantarum – Knocking down the histamine levels and packing your body with amazing properties that can improve your overall health, this strain is definitely welcome for those that are intolerant to histamine.

However, you need to be extremely careful when supplementing your diet with probiotics. The study and research on this topic are pretty limited at this point, but according to many scientists, there are certain probiotics strains that can, in fact, produce histamine. To keep your health and diet in check, you need to make sure not to take such probiotic strains:

Lactobacillus Reuteri – Besides the fact that this probiotic is a powerful antioxidant that can knock down IBS (Irritable Bowel Syndrome) it may not be so beneficial for those with histamine intolerance as it can actually produce histamine.

Lactobacillus Helveticus – This is another probiotic strain that produces histamine. Besides its amazing benefits, if you are suffering from histamine intolerance, make sure that your supplements do not contain this strain.

Lactobacillus Casei – It may be a great allergy reliever and an amazing supporter of the proper liver functioning, but lactobacillus casei can aggravate the symptoms of histamine intolerance. Make sure not to include it in your diet.

Lactobacillus Bularicus – Another probiotic strain that you need to stay away from in order to keep your gut balanced and the side effects at bay.

DAO Enzymes

A DAO supplement is great for those with DAO deficiency, as well as for a short-term relief of the symptoms, as it promotes histamine clearance. There are tons of these supplements on the market so it may be challenging to pick the right one. Ask your doctor to prescribe you the best. I, personally, find HistamAid88 to be quite helpful.

Quercetin

Its bioflavonoids help fight inflammation and can constrain the release of the histamine from the mast cells. Most people have found that taking about 400 to 600 mg three times a day is most beneficial, however, this is something that you need to discuss with your doctor. Know that quercetin works best when combined with bromelain.

Luteolin

This flavone will not only help you fight off inflammation (which is basically the heart of histamine intolerance), but it will also slow down the activity of the mast cells that is in charge of releasing histamine. A dose of 100 mg, two times a day, is what works for the majority of histamine intolerant individuals.

Silibinin

Silibinin, comes from milk thistle, and is also capable of preventing histamine release. Plus, silibinin also prevents the release of other inflammatory cytokines. Besides, this compound will also stimulate your liver to function more efficiently. Herb Pharm Milk Thistle contains silibinin and it has proven to be very effective amongst people with histamine intolerance.

Vitamin C

Being one of the most powerful antioxidants, vitamin C can also purge the inflammatory compounds, such as histamine from your blood. In addition, it will also increase your DAO enzymes. Make sure not to start with a large dose as that can cause loose stools.

Histamine Elimination 6-Week Meal Plan

Now that you know what should and shouldn't be eaten, it is time for you to take a look at the ultimate 6-week elimination meal plan. Make sure to track your progress carefully during these six weeks and take notice of any change and improvements in the symptoms, and the way you feel, in general.

Again, please discuss the elimination of histamine with your doctor before removing histamine-rich foods from your kitchen and starting this histamine elimination meal plan. Most people start anywhere from one to three months to be able to reverse their condition. If your doctor feels that you need more than 6 weeks to get rid of the excess histamine levels from your body, you can simply repeat this meal plan for another six weeks (if it is not too boring for you, of course). However, I have balanced and carefully created this meal plan, and I highly suggest that, should you need more weeks of histamine elimination, you roll up your sleeves and get creative with meal planning.

WEEK 1

Day 1:

Breakfast:

2 hard-boiled Eggs
1 gluten-free and yeast-free Flatbread
1 tbsp. Cream Cheese
½ cup grated Carrots, Cabbage, and Beets
½ glass of allowed Fruit Juice

Snack 1:

½ cup Pretzels
½ cup Mango Chunks

Lunch:

1 cup creamy Soup with Broccoli, Cauliflower, and Mozzarella Cheese
2 tbsp. gluten-free and yeast-free Croutons
½ cup shredded Cucumber, Ricotta, Mint, and Basil Salad, drizzled with Olive Oil
1 Apple

Snack 2:

1 gluten-free and yeast-free Vanilla Muffin
1 glass of Hemp Milk

Dinner:

6-ounce Beef Steak
5 Asparagus Spears
½ cup mashed Potatoes
2 tbsp sautéed Mushrooms
½ glass of fresh Pomegranate Juice

Day 2:

Breakfast:

2 Potato Fritters
2 tbsp Cottage Cheese
½ cup chopped allowed Veggies
1 Pear

Snack 1:

1 cup Kale Chips
½ cup Pomegranate Molasses
1 Apricot

Lunch:

1 cup of Clean Chicken Soup
½ gluten-free and yeast-free
Flatbread
1 cup Quinoa, Kale, Carrot,
Parsley, and Mozzarella Salad

Snack 2:

1 piece of Blueberry Cobbler
made with Coconut Flour
1 glass of Coconut Milk

Dinner:

1 grilled fresh-caught Cod
Fillet
½ cup cooked Rice
½ cup steamed Brussels
Sprouts
2 scoops of Ice Cream made
with allowed ingredients

Day 3:

Breakfast:

2 slices of gluten-free and
yeast-free Bread
3 tbsp. Applesauce
1 glass of Coconut Milk

Snack 1:

3 tbsp. anti-histamine
Hummus (made with pureed
Cauliflower, olive oil,
turmeric, paprika, and garlic)
2 Baby Carrots
3 gluten-free Crackers
2 Celery Sticks

Lunch:

1 cup Fish Stew made with
fresh-caught cod or tilapia and
allowed veggies
½ gluten-free, yeast-free
Flatbread
1/2 cup grated Beets drizzled
with Olive Oil

Snack 2:

1 cup Rice Pudding made with
Coconut Milk

Dinner:

1 Lamb Chop, cooked
4 White Button Mushrooms,
grilled
½ cup mashed Potatoes
½ cup Cucumber, Mint, and
Arugula Salad topped with 1
ounce Mozzarella
1 cup Cherries

Day 4:

Breakfast:

½ cup cooked Millet
½ cup Coconut Milk
1 tbsp. Applesauce
¼ cup Blueberries
¼ cup pureed Mango

Snack 1:

2 Rice Cakes
1 cup Cherries

Lunch:

Turkey Sandwich made with 2 slices of gluten-free and yeast-free Bread, 3 ounces cooked and shredded Turkey, 1 tbsp. Cream Cheese, 1 Lettuce Leaf, 1/4 Cucumber, sliced. 2 tbsp. shredded Red Cabbage
1 Peach

Snack 2:

1 cup Zucchini Chips
1 glass of allowed Veggie Juice
1 Apricot

Dinner:

1 5-ounce Tilapia Fillet, baked
½ cup sweet Potato cubes, baked
1 Carrot, baked
1 cup Salad with Bell Peppers, Cucumbers, Lettuce, Onions, and Mozzarella
½ cup Pomegranate Molasses

Day 5:

Breakfast:

2 pieces of French toast made with gluten-free and yeast-free Bread, Eggs, and Coconut Milk
¼ cup Blackberries
2 tbsp. Blueberries
2 tbsp. Black Currants
2 tbsp. Cream Cheese
1 glass of Coconut Milk

Snack 1:

½ cup Pretzels
1 Pear
½ glass of allowed Fruit Juice

Lunch:

Chicken Quinoa Bowl (1/2 cup cooked Quinoa, 3 ounces cooked and shredded chicken, a handful of basil, 1 tbsp. Cottage Cheese, 1 ounce Mozzarella Cheese, ½ grated Carrot)
1 piece of allowed fruit

Snack 2:

1 cup of Apple Chips
1 tbsp. Organic and Unsweetened Applesauce

Dinner:

1 cup of Beef Stew, made with allowed ingredients
1 piece of gluten-free and yeast-free Bread
1 cup Cabbage, Beet, and Carrot salad
2 scoops of Ice Cream, made with allowed ingredients

Day 6:

Breakfast:

3 Cauliflower and Egg Fritters
2 tbsp. Cream Cheese
1 Carrot
1/3 cup shredded Cabbage, drizzled with some olive oil
1 Apple

Snack 1:

1 cup of Rice Pudding made with Dairy-Free Milk

Lunch:

1 cup of clean Vegetable Soup
1 slice of gluten-free and yeast-free Bread
1 cup of Mint, Watercress, Tarragon, Zucchini, and Cucumber Salad
1 ounce Mozzarella Cheese
1 Peach

Snack 2:

1 cup of Popcorn
½ cup Pomegranate Molasses

Dinner:

1 cup of cooked Spaghetti
4 Beef Meatballs

¼ cup white sauce made with mashed cauliflower and allowed cheese
1 glass of allowed Fruit Juice

Day 7:

Breakfast:

¾ cup cooked Oatmeal
½ cup Coconut Milk
2 tbsp. Pomegranate Molasses
1 tbsp. Applesauce
½ Peach, cut into chunks

Snack 1:

1 cup Watermelon Chunks
2 gluten-free Crackers
1 tbsp. Cream Cheese

Lunch:

Beef Sandwich made with two slices of gluten-free and yeast-free Bread, 3 ounces of cooked and shredded Beef, 1 Lettuce leaf, and 1 tbsp. Ricotta Cheese, ½ grated Carrot, and chopped tarragon
A glass of allowed Fruit Juice

Snack 2:

2 tbsp. Anti-Histamine Hummus (made with mashed broccoli, olive oil, herbs, and cheese)
2 Baby Carrots
½ Cucumber, cut into strips

Dinner:

½ cup cooked Quinoa
4-ounce grilled Chicken
4 steamed Asparagus Spears
1 ounce Mozzarella Cheese
2 scoops of Ice Cream made with allowed ingredients

WEEK 2

Day 1

Breakfast:

2 Pancakes made with gluten-free flour such as Coconut Flour

2 tbsp. Cream Cheese
½ cup mushed allowed Fruit
½ glass of Coconut Milk

Snack 1:

½ cup Roasted Veggies
topped with 2 Mozzarella
Slices

Lunch:

1 cup of Creamy Veggie Soup
½ gluten-free Flat Bread
4 ounces grilled Salmon
½ cup Cherries

Snack 2:

½ cup of Pretzels
1 tbsp. Pure Organic and
Unsweetened Applesauce

Dinner:

1 Bell Pepper stuffed with 2
tbsp. cooked Rice, 3 tbsp.
minced Beef, some grated
Carrot, grated Zucchini, and ½
tbsp. chopped Onion

1/2 gluten-free Flat Bread
A glass of allowed Fruit Juice

Day 2:

Breakfast:

½ Bagel
1 tbsp. Organic and
Unsweetened Applesauce
1 glass of Coconut Milk
1 apple

Snack 1:

1 hard-boiled Egg

Lunch:

½ cup steamed veggies such
as Broccoli, Carrots, and
Cauliflower
½ cup mashed Potatoes
4-ounces grilled Chicken
A handful of steamed Kale
Leaves drizzled with olive Oil
1 Peach

Snack 2:

2 Rice Cakes

54

½ cup Mango Chunks

Dinner:

1 piece of Lasagna made with
gluten-free pasta, gluten-free
and dairy-free béchamel
sauce, minced beef, and
mozzarella cheese
1 small piece of Garlic Bread
(baked bread topped with
garlic powder and fresh
herbs)
A handful of Black Currants

Day 3:

Breakfast:

½ cup cooked Polenta
1 ounce Mozzarella Cheese
½ cup sautéed Veggies
1 cup Blackberries

Snack 1:

1 plain gluten-free Muffin
½ glass of Almond Milk

Lunch:

Turkey Wrap made with
gluten-free wrap, 3 ounces

cooked Turkey meat, and 2
tbsp. chopped fresh veggies, 1
tbsp. Cottage Cheese
1 Apple

Snack 2:

3 gluten-free crackers
1 cup fruit Smoothie made
with allowed ingredients

Dinner:

1 Chicken Drumstick
½ cup cooked Rice
1 cup Leafy Green Salad
drizzled with Olive Oil
½ glass of Coconut Milk

Day 4:

Breakfast:

2 Hardboiled Eggs
1 slice of gluten-free and
yeast-free Bread
A handful of allowed chopped
Veggies
1 ounce of allowed Cheese
½ cup Pomegranate Molasses

Snack 1:

1 piece of Peach Cobbler made
with allowed ingredients
1 glass of Hemp Milk

Lunch:

1 cup of Chicken Soup
2 tbsp. of gluten-free Croutons
½ cup cooked quinoa topped
with 1 ounce Mozzarella
Cheese
1 Apricot

Snack 2:

1 piece of toasted gluten-free
and yeast-free Bread, topped
with 1 tbsp. allowed Fruit Jam

Dinner:

4 ounces of cooked Lamb
Meat
½ Sweet Potato, roasted
½ cup of steamed Broccoli
1 Carrot, steamed
4 Asparagus Spears, steamed
½ glass of allowed Fruit Juice

Day 5:

Breakfast:

2 Potato Latkes
2 tbsp. Cream Cheese
1 handful of fresh Leafy
Greens drizzled with Olive Oil
½ glass of Coconut Milk

Snack 1:

1 Apple
1 tbsp. Pure Organic and
Unsweetened Applesauce

Lunch:

1 gluten-free Tortilla
3 ounces Pulled Pork
2 Lettuce Leaves, shredded
3 Onion Rings
1 tbsp. Ricotta Cheese
1 Peach

Snack 2:

1 cup of smoothie made with Greens and allowed Fruit

Dinner:

1 cup cooked Penne Pasta
½ cup Cauliflower and Cheese Sauce
2 Asparagus Spears, roasted and chopped
2 Artichoke Hearts
½ cup Cherries

Day 6:

Breakfast:

2 Gluten-Free Pancakes
¼ cup Cherries
1 tbsp. Applesauce
1 glass of Coconut Milk
½ Apple

Snack 1:

½ cup Pretzels
2 Apricots

Lunch:

A handful of Greens
½ cup cooked Rice
4 ounces of grilled Cod
½ glass of allowed Fruit Juice

Snack 2:

2 tbsp. Cream Cheese
2 gluten-free Crackers
2 baby Carrots
¼ Cucumber, cut into strips

Dinner:

1 Zucchini, spiralized
3 ounces minced Beef, cooked with 1 tbsp. chopped onion and ½ Garlic Clove minced
¼ cup of mashed Cauliflower and Cheese Pasta Sauce
½ cup Pomegranate Molasses

Day 7:

Breakfast:

½ cup cooked Oats
¼ cup mashed allowed Fruit
½ glass of Coconut Milk

2 tbsp. Coconut Shavings
1 tsp. Honey, optional

2 Asparagus Spears, steamed

Snack 1:

1 cup Kale Chips
1 Peach

Lunch:

½ cup cooked Rice
2 tbsp. sautéed Mushrooms
1 ounce Mozzarella Cheese
½ cup steamed Broccoli
Florets

Snack 2:

1 tbsp. Organic and
Unsweetened Applesauce
1 Rice Cake
½ cup Cantaloupe Chunks

Dinner:

5 ounces of Beef Steak
½ cup cooked Polenta
½ cup of Watercress, Lettuce,
and Tarragon Salad, drizzled
with Olive Oil
1 Carrot, steamed

WEEK 3

Day 1:

Breakfast:

1 Hardboiled Egg
1 slice of gluten-free and
yeast-free Bread
½ cup of steamed chopped
Veggies
1 ounce Mozzarella Cheese
½ Apple

Snack 1:

3 gluten-free Biscuits
1 tbsp. allowed Fruit Jam
½ glass of Dairy-Free Milk

Lunch:

½ Zucchini, roasted and
topped with 2 slices of
Mozzarella Cheese
4 ounces of cooked Salmon
A handful of allowed Greens
drizzled with Olive Oil
½ cup Cherries

Snack 2:

½ cup Pretzels
1 tbsp. Organic and
Unsweetened Applesauce

Dinner:

1 cup of Chicken Stew
½ cup gluten-free Flatbread
1 cup of Lettuce, Cucumber,
Carrot, and Onion Salad with
Olive Oil
½ cup Watermelon Chunks

Day 2:

Breakfast:

½ cup cooked Quinoa
2 tbsp. caramelized Onions
1 tbsp. Cottage Cheese
½ cup shredded cabbage
drizzled with Olive Oil
½ cup sated Veggies
1 glass of allowed Fruit Juice

Snack 1:

1 tbsp. Organic and
Unsweetened Applesauce
3 gluten-free Biscuits
1 glass of Coconut Milk

Lunch:

4 ounces cooked Meat by
choice
1 cup mashed Potatoes
A handful of Greens
1/3 cup grated Beets drizzled
with Olive Oil
1 Peach

Snack 2:

½ cup Cantaloupe Chunks
2 tbsp. Coconut Shavings
1 tsp Honey
2 tbsp. Pomegranate Molasses

Dinner:

1 cup cooked Rice Noodles
3 ounces steamed and
shredded Fish
1 ounce Mozzarella Cheese
1 grated Carrot
¼ cup mashed Cauliflower
2 scoops Ice Cream made with
allowed ingredients

Day 3:

Breakfast:

2 scrambled Eggs
1 tbsp. sautéed Onions
1 tbsp. Cream Cheese
1 slice of gluten-free and
yeast-free Bread
A handful of allowed Greens
A handful of Black Currants

Snack 1:

2 Rice Cakes
1 glass of Almond Milk

Lunch:

1 cup of Creamy Potato and
Cheese Soup
2 tbsp. gluten-free Croutons
1 cup allowed Salad by choice
½ cup Green Grapes

Snack 2:

6 Asparagus Spears roasted
with garlic powder and
gluten-free breadcrumbs
2 tbsp. Ricotta Cheese
½ glass of allowed Fruit Juice

Dinner:

1 5-ounce Pork Chop

1 tbsp. caramelized Onions
½ cup cooked Polenta
1 cup of salad with Cucumber,
Mint, Parsley, Watercress and
Cottage Cheese

Day 4:

Breakfast:

2 Turkey and Zucchini
Breakfast Fritters made with
3 ounces of ground Turkey
Meat, ½ grated Zucchini,
herbs, chopped Spring Onion
and 1 Egg
1 ounce Mozzarella Cheese
½ gluten-free Tortilla
A glass of allowed Fruit Juice

Snack 1:

1 cup of Onion Rings made
with eggs and gluten-free
flour
1 tbsp. Ricotta Cheese

Lunch:

4 Meatballs
1 cup cooked Rice Noodles
1 cup of Salad by choice

½ cup Watermelon Chunks

Snack 2:

1 piece of Apple Pie made
with allowed ingredients
1 glass of Diary-Free Milk

Dinner:

1 cup mashed Potatoes
1 Carrot, sautéed
½ cup Broccoli, sautéed
4 Artichoke Hearts, sautéed
2 ounces Mozzarella Cheese
A handful of allowed Greens
drizzled with Olive Oil
1 cup Cherries

Day 5:

Breakfast:

2 Hardboiled Eggs
1 slice of gluten-free and
yeast-free Bread
2 slices of Mozzarella Cheese
1 tbsp. caramelized Onions
1 Apple

Snack 1:

1 cup Popcorn

½ cup Mango Chunks

Lunch:

½ cup cooked Quinoa
½ cup steamed Brussel
Sprouts
1 tbsp. Ricotta Cheese
¼ small Onion, sliced
1 tbsp. gluten-free
Breadcrumbs
½ cup Pomegranate Molasses

Snack 2:

1 Plain Muffin
½ glass of Coconut Milk

Dinner:

5 ounces of cooked Ground
Beef with some chopped
Onion and minced Garlic
1 cup of cooked Pasta
½ cup of mashed Cauliflower
and Cheese White Pasta Sauce
A handful of allowed Greens
1 Peach

Day 6:

Breakfast:

2/3 cup cooked Oatmeal
2 tbsp. Coconut Shavings
2 tbsp. Black Currants
2 tbsp. Applesauce
½ cup of Coconut Milk

Snack 1:

1 cup French Fries
1 tbsp. Ricotta Cheese

Lunch:

1 cup of clean Veggie Soup
½ slice of gluten-free and
yeast-free Bread
4-ounce grilled Chicken
½ cup mashed Potatoes

Snack 1:

1 cup Watermelon Chunks
½ cup Pretzels

Dinner:

1 gluten-free Hamburger Bun
1 Veggie Pattie made with
Broccoli, Cauliflower,

Zucchini, Onions, Herbs, Egg, and Breadcrumbs
1 Lettuce Leaf
1 tbsp. Cream Cheese
½ grated Carrot drizzled with some Olive Oil
½ cup Cherries

Day 7:

Breakfast:

2 gluten-free Pancakes
2 tbsp. Organic and Unsweetened Applesauce
1 glass of Coconut Milk

Snack 1:

1 cup Zucchini Chips
1 cup Pomegranate Molasses

Lunch:

½ cup cooked Quinoa
1 shredded Apple
2 tbsp. Red Currants
2 tbsp. Blueberries
2 tbsp. Coconut Shavings
1 tsp Honey

Snack 2:

1 plain Muffin
1 glass of allowed Juice

Dinner:

5 ounces grilled Salmon
4 Asparagus spears, steamed
A handful of Greens drizzled with Olive Oil
½ cup mashed Potatoes
2 scoops of Ice Cream made with allowed ingredients

WEEK 4

Day 1:

Breakfast:

1 slice of Frittata made with allowed Vegetables
1 slice of gluten-free and yeast-free Bread
1 ounce Mozzarella Cheese
½ Apple

Snack 1:

1 cup Pretzels
1 Apricot

Lunch:

1 cup of Beef and Rice Noodle Soup
1 cup of Salad made with Cucumber, Carrot, Lettuce, Kale, and drizzled with Olive Oil
1 Apple

Snack 2:

1 piece of Pumpkin Pie
1 glass of Diary-Free Milk

Dinner:

1 Chicken Drumstick and 1 Chicken Thigh (no more than 6 ounces of meat in total)
½ cup cooked Rice
½ cup steamed allowed Veggies
1/3 cup grated Beets drizzled with Olive Oil
1 Peach

Day 2:

Breakfast:

½ cup cooked Oats
1 Apple, shredded
¼ cup mashed Mango
2 tbsp. Pomegranate Molasses
1 gluten-free Biscuit, crumbed
1 tbsp. Coconut Shavings
½ glass of Coconut Milk

Snack 1:

1 cup of allowed Fruit Smoothie
½ cup Kale Chips

Lunch:

4 ounces of cooked Salmon
1 medium Potato, boiled
2 Mozzarella Slices
½ Cucumber
½ cup shredded Cabbage
drizzled with Olive Oil
½ cup Cherries

Snack 2:

2 tbsp. Cream Cheese
2 Baby Carrots
3 gluten-free Crackers
½ Bell Pepper, cut into strips

Dinner:

1 Hamburger Bun
4 ounces of Pulled Pork
½ cup Salad by your choice
(allowed ingredients only)
1 scoop of allowed Ice Cream

Day 3:

Breakfast:

1 Hardboiled Egg
1 slice of gluten-free and
yeast-free Bread

½ cup sautéed Veggies
1 tbsp. Ricotta Cheese
A handful of Greens
1 Peach

Snack 1:

1 serving of Apple Crumb
made with allowed
ingredients
1 glass of Dairy-Free Milk

Lunch:

1 cup of Clean Vegetable Soup
½ cup cooked Rice
4 ounces grilled Salmon
A handful of Greens drizzled
with Olive Oil

Snack 2:

1 cup Kale Chips
1 cup Cherries

Dinner:
1 cup cooked Pasta
3 ounces cooked and
Shredded Chicken
½ cup sautéed allowed
Vegetables

1 tbsp. Cottage Cheese
½ cup Mango Chunks

Day 4:

Breakfast:

2 gluten-free Pancakes
2 tbsp. Cream Cheese
½ cup mix of sautéed Onions,
Kale, Broccoli, and Carrots
1 Peach

Snack 1:

1 cup Baked Sweet Potato
Chips sprinkled with
Turmeric
1 glass of allowed Fruit Juice

Lunch:

1 gluten-free Wrap
4-ounce of grilled Chicken,
sliced
A handful of Arugula
1 tbsp. Riccota Cheese
1/3 cup shredded Cabbage
and Beets drizzled with Olive
Oil
½ cup Pomegranate Molasses

Snack 2:

1 Apple
1 tbsp. Organic and
Unsweetened Applesauce
½ glass of Coconut Milk

Dinner:

1/2 cup Mashed Potatoes
1 cup of Beef Bourguignon,
made with allowed
ingredients
1 cup of Cucumber,
Watercress, Peppermint, and
Lettuce Salad drizzled with
Olive Oil
1 scoop of Ice Cream made
with allowed ingredients

Day 5:

Breakfast:

1 gluten-free Plain Muffin
1 tbsp. Organic and
Unsweetened Applesauce
1 Apple
1 glass of Coconut Milk

Snack 1:

2 Rice Cakes
1 Peach

Lunch:

1 cup of Chicken and Noodle
Soup
1 cup of allowed Salad by
choice
2 slices of Garlic Bread
(French loaf)
½ cup Pomegranate Molasses

Snack 2:

1 cup Pretzels
½ cup Blackberries

Dinner:

1 cup cooked Spaghetti
¼ cup mashed Cauliflower
and Cheese Pasta Sauce
4 Meatballs
½ cup allowed Greens
drizzled with Olive Oil
½ cup Watermelon Chunks

Day 6:

Breakfast:

2 Hardboiled Eggs
1 slice of gluten-free and
yeast-free Bread
1 ounce Mozzarella Cheese
1 Spring Onion
1/3 cup grated Beets drizzled
with Olive Oil

Snack 1:

1 Apple
1 tbsp. Organic and
Unsweetened Applesauce
½ glass of Coconut Milk

Lunch:

1 gluten-free Tortilla
2 ounces cooked and
shredded Fish
A handful of allowed Greens
1 tbsp. Cottage Cheese
1 Pear

Snack 2:

1 cup Zucchini Chips
½ cup Cherries

Dinner:

5-ounce Beef Steak

1 cup mashed Potatoes
4 Artichoke Hearts Steamed
1 Carrot, steamed
A handful of Black Currants

Day 7:

Breakfast:

2/3 cup cooked Millet
2 tbsp. Coconut Shavings
1 tsp. Honey
2 tbsp. Blueberries
1 tbsp. Applesauce, optional
½ glass of Coconut Milk

Snack 1:

1 tbsp. Cream Cheese
2 gluten-free Crackers
2 Baby Carrots
½ glass allowed Fruit Juice

Lunch:

1 cup of Creamy Veggie Soup
2 slices of Garlic Bread
(French loaf)
1 cup of allowed Salad by
choice drizzled with Olive Oil
1 ounce Mozzarella Cheese

Snack 2:

1 piece of Apple Pie
½ glass of Dairy-Free Milk

Dinner:

6-ounce Lamb Chopped
2 tbsp. Caramelized Onions
½ cup cooked Polenta
½ cup steamed allowed
Veggies by choice
2 scoops of Ice Cream made
with allowed ingredients

WEEK 5

Day 1:

Breakfast:

2 scrambled Eggs
½ gluten-free Bagel
1 tbsp. Cream Cheese
2 tbsp. sautéed Mushrooms
½ cup Pomegranate Molasses

Snack 1:

1 cup Apple chips drizzled
with 1 tsp. of Honey
1 Rice Cake

Lunch:

1/2 cup cooked Quinoa
½ cup sautéed allowed
Veggies
1 ounces allowed Cheese
½ cup Mango Chunks

Snack 1:

1 plain gluten-free Muffin
1 glass of Coconut Milk

Dinner:

1 cup of Chicken Stew
1 slice of gluten-free and
yeast-free Bread
1 cup of allowed Salad by
choice
½ cup Cantaloupe Chunks

Day 2:

Breakfast:

2 slices of gluten-free and
yeast-free Bread, toasted
2 tbsp. allowed Fruit Jam
1 cup of Dairy Free Milk

Snack 1:

1 cup of Popcorn
1 Peach

Lunch:

1 cup of Clean Veggie Soup
½ cup cooked Rice
4 ounces cooked Cod
2 tbsp. caramelized Onion

1 ounce Mozzarella Cheese

Snack 1:

1 cup of French Fries topped with 1 ounce of Mozzarella Cheese and microwaved until melted
½ glass of allowed Fruit Juice

Snack 2:

1 cup of Zucchini Chips
1 Smoothie made with 1 Apple, a handful of Kale, 2 tbsp. Coconut Shavings, ½ cup Mango Chunks, and ½ cup Coconut Milk

Lunch:

1 cup of Nettle Soup
½ gluten-free Flat Bread
1 cup Watermelon Chunks

Dinner:

4 ounces of cooked Turkey Meat
1 gluten-free Wrap
½ cup chopped allowed Veggies
1 ounce of allowed Cheese
¼ cup mashed allowed Fruit
1 scoop of Vanilla Ice Cream made with Dairy-Free Milk

Snack 2:

1 piece of Peach Cobbler
1 glass of Coconut Milk

Dinner:

2 Chicken Drumsticks
½ cup mashed Cauliflower and Broccoli
A handful of Greens drizzled with Olive Oil
2 tbsp. caramelized Onions
1 cup Cherries

Day 3:

Breakfast:

1 piece of Quiche made with allowed ingredients
½ gluten-free Bagel
1 tbsp. Curd Cheese
½ Apple

Day 4:

Breakfast:

½ cup cooked Quinoa
½ cup Almond Milk
1 tbsp. Organic and
Unsweetened Applesauce
1 Apple, grated
1 tbsp. Pomegranate Molasses

Snack 1:

1 cup Onion Rings made with
Eggs and gluten-free Flour
1 ounce allowed Cheese
½ glass of allowed Fruit Juice

Lunch:

1 cup cooked Rice
2 tbsp. caramelized Onions
1 ounce Mozzarella Cheese
3 ounces cooked and
shredded Turkey Meat
A handful of Greens drizzled
with Olive Oil

Snack 2:

1 piece of Cake made with
allowed Ingredients
½ cup Coconut Milk

Dinner:

1 gluten-free Hamburger Bun
1 4-ounce Beef Pattie
¼ cup shredded Cabbage and
Carrot drizzled with Olive Oil
1 Lettuce Leaf
1 Mozzarella Slice

Day 5:

Breakfast:

1 Hardboiled Egg
½ Bagel
2 slices Mozzarella Cheese
½ cups sautéed Onions,
Carrots, Zucchini, and
chopped Asparagus
½ glass allowed Fruit Juice

Snack 1:

½ cup Pretzels

Lunch:

Organic and Unsweetened Applesauce and Berry Jelly Sandwich made with 2 slices of gluten-free and yeast-free Bread, 1 tbsp. Applesauce and 1 tbsp Berry Jelly
½ glass Coconut Milk

1 Peach

Snack 1:

1 piece of Apple Pie
½ glass of Coconut Milk

Snack 2:

1 cup Kale Chips
1 cup allowed Fruit Chunks

Lunch:

1 gluten-free Hamburger Bun
4-ounce Turkey and Zucchini Pattie
1 tbsp. Ricotta Cheese
A handful of Greens drizzled with Olive Oil
1 Kiwi Fruit

Dinner:

5-ounce Grilled Chicken Breast
½ cup mashed Potatoes
1 steamed Carrot
3 steamed Artichoke Hearts
1 slice of Garlic Bread (French loaf)
½ cup Pomegranate Molasses

Snack 1:

1 cup Rice Pudding made with Coconut Milk

Dinner:

1 cup of Fish Stew
1 slice of gluten-free and yeast-free Bread
1 cup of Cucumber, Watercress, Lettuce, and Mint Salad topped with 1 ounce of allowed Cheese
½ cup Pomegranate Molasses

Day 6:

Breakfast:

2 Potato Latkes
2 tbsp. Cream Cheese
1 cup of chopped allowed Veggies

1 cup grated Apple
1 tsp Honey

Day 7:

Breakfast:

2 scrambled Eggs
½ cup sautéed allowed
Veggies
1 gluten-free English Muffin
1 ounce of allowed Cheese
1 Peach

Dinner:

4-ounces baked and battered
Tilapia (with Eggs and
Coconut Flour)
½ cup cooked Rice
½ cup steamed Veggies
2 scoops of Ice Cream made
with allowed Ingredients

Snack 1:

½ cup Pretzels
1 tbsp. Organic and
Unsweetened Applesauce

Lunch:

1 cup mashed Potatoes
4 ounces cooked and
Shredded Chicken
A handful of allowed Greens
drizzled with Olive Oil
1 slice Garlic Bread (French
Loaf)
½ cup Watermelon Chunks

Snack 2:

2 tbsp. Coconut Shavings
2 tbsp. Black Currants

WEEK 6

Day 1:

Breakfast:

2 Hardboiled Eggs
1 slice of gluten-free and yeast-free Bread
1 tbsp. Cream Cheese
1 glass of Rice Milk

Snack 1:

A handful of Pretzels
1 cup of cantaloupe Cubes

Lunch:

1 cup Onion Soup
2 tbsp. gluten-free Croutons
1 cup Cucumber, Parsley, and Olive Oil Salad
1 ounce Mozzarella Cheese
1 Apple

Snack 2:

1 cup Sweet Potato Chips
2 Baby Carrots

1 glass of allowed Fruit Juice

Dinner:

½ cup cooked Rice
4 ounces of Beef Steak
4 Asparagus Spears, steamed
2 tbsp. caramelized Onions
1 peach

Day 2:

Breakfast:

1 gluten-free Bagel
2 tbsp. allowed Fruit Jam
1 Apricot

Snack 1:

3 Rice Cookies
1 glass of Almond Milk

Lunch:

1 cup Leafy Green Salad (not spinach)
4 ounces cooked Turkey Meat
½ cup mashed Potatoes
A handful of Blackberries

Snack 2:

1 cup Watermelon Chunks
2 ounces allowed Cheese

Dinner:

1 cup cooked gluten-free
Pasta
1 cup sautéed allowed Veggies
2 scoops of Ice Cream made
with allowed ingredients

Day 3:

Breakfast:

2 scrambled Eggs
1 slice of gluten-free and
yeast-free Bread, toasted
1 tbsp. Cottage Cheese
2 tbsp. caramelized Onions
3 Kale Leaves, sautéed

Snack 1:

1 cup of allowed Fruit Chunks
drizzled with 1 tsp. Honey

Lunch:

1 cup of clean Veggie Soup
½ cup cooked Quinoa
3 ounces cooked and
Shredded Chicken
1 cup Salad (Onion, Carrot,
Cucumber, Chard, Holy Basil,
Olive Oil)

Snack 2:

1 gluten-free Plain Muffin
1 tbsp. Organic and
Unsweetened Applesauce

Dinner:

1 5-ounce fillet of Salmon
1 Large Potato, baked
4 Artichoke Hearts, steamed
1 ounce Mozzarella Cheese
2 Apricots

Day 4:

Breakfast:

1 cup Rice Krispies
1 cup Coconut Milk
2 tbsp. Blueberries
5 Blackberries

Snack 1:

2 Baby Carrots
½ Cucumber, cut into strips
½ Bell Pepper, cut into strips
2 ounces Cottage Cheese

Lunch:

1 cup Clean Chicken Soup
1 slice of gluten-free Bread
½ cup sautéed Chards and
Kale
2 Peach

Snack 2:

1 cup Popcorn
1 scoop of Ice Cream made
with allowed ingredients

Dinner:

4 ounces grilled Chicken
Breast
½ cup cooked Rice
½ cup cooked Broccoli Florets
2 slices Mozzarella Cheese
1 glass of allowed Fruit Juice

Day 5:

Breakfast:

Cheese and Mushroom Omelet
(2 Eggs, 1 ½ ounces Young
Cheese, 2 sliced Mushrooms)
1 slice of gluten-free and
yeast-free Bread
½ cup Mango Chunks

Snack 1:

½ cup Pretzels
½ cup allowed Fruit Chunks

Lunch:

1 cup cooked quinoa
1 ounce Mozzarella Cheese
½ cup steamed allowed
Veggies
2 tbsp. chopped Parsley

Snack 2:

1 cup of Smoothie with
allowed ingredients:

Dinner:

5 ounces Pulled Pork
½ cup Mashed Potatoes
4 steamed Asparagus Spears
2 tbsp. Caramelized Onions
A handful of Black Currants

Day 6:

Breakfast:

½ cup cooked Millet
½ cup Hemp Milk
½ Apple
¼ cu Blueberries

Snack 1:

½ cup Pomegranate Molasses
½ Apple
1 tbsp. Organic and
Unsweetened Applesauce

Lunch:

1 gluten-free Hamburger Bun
3-ounce Beef Pattie
½ cup allowed Salad by choice
½ cup Green Grapes

Snack 2:

½ cup sliced allowed Veggies
2 tbsp. Cream Cheese
1 tsp. Honey, optional

Dinner:

1 cup cooked gluten-free
Pasta
3 ounces cooked and
shredded Turkey
2 tbsp. Caramelized Onions
4 Broccoli Florets, steamed
1 ½ ounce Mozzarella Cheese
1 Peach

Day 7:

Breakfast:

1 cup of gluten-free Granola
1 cup Coconut Milk
¼ cup Mango Chunks

Snack 1:

½ Zucchini topped with 1
ounce of Mozzarella Cheese
and baked

Lunch:

Organic and Unsweetened
Applesauce and Jelly
Sandwich, gluten-free and
made with allowed
ingredients

Snack 2:

1 cup Cherries
2 tbsp. Ricotta Cheese

Dinner:

Chicken Drumstick and Thigh
(about 6 ounces meat in total)
½ cup mashed Potatoes
1 slice of Garlic Bread (French
Loaf)
A handful of Greens drizzled
with Olive Oil
½ cup Pomegranate Molasses

Talk to Your Doctor!

I hope that this book was able to help you clear the confusion about histamine intolerance, as well as to determine what the best approach for treating your condition is.

The next step is to simply discuss your plan with your doctor and start the histamine elimination diet the right way. Many people have lowered their histamine levels with this diet, so why can't you?

One last thing... If you enjoyed this book, you can help me tremendously by leaving a review on Amazon. You have no idea how much this would help.

I also want to give you a chance to win a **$200.00 Amazon Gift Card** as a thank-you for reading this book.

All I ask is that you give me some feedback! You can also copy/paste your *Amazon* or *Goodreads review* and this will also count.

Your opinion is valuable to me. It will only take a minute of your time to let me know what you like and what you didn't like about this book. The hardest part is deciding how to spend the two hundred dollars! Just follow this link.

reviewers.win/antihistamine

[Page intentionally left blank]

Made in United States
Orlando, FL
30 November 2021

10975746R00049